FIBROMYALGIA

SIMPLE INSTRUCTIONS FOR TREATING

FIBROMYALGIA

DR. MARSH NEAL

Contents

CHAPTER ONE

INTRODUCTION

Fibromyalgia motives ache on your muscles and joints sooner or later of your body. It can additionally make you experience fatigued and purpose intellectual signs and symptoms and symptoms like memory issues. Experts don't understand what causes fibromyalgia — and there's no treatment for it — however a healthcare organisation will assist you find treatments to govern your signs and signs.

Fibromyalgia is an extended-term (chronic) health condition that reasons pain and tenderness throughout your frame. It reasons musculoskeletal pain and fatigue.

Humans with fibromyalgia typically experience signs and symptoms and symptoms that come and cross during periods referred to as flare-ups. Sometimes, it can revel in exhausting and challenging to navigate living with fibromyalgia. The peaks and valleys among feeling suitable and unexpectedly having a flare-up of symptoms and signs and symptoms can sense overwhelming. Fibromyalgia is real, and so is how you experience.

Specialists don't recognise what reasons fibromyalgia, however studies have located that sure health conditions, strain and distinctive modifications for your life might also trigger it. You is probably much more likely to extend fibromyalgia if one in all your organic parents has it.

Any new pain on your body is frequently the first sign of fibromyalgia — specifically in your muscle mass. Accept as true with your instincts and concentrate in your frame. Go to a healthcare corporation in case you're experiencing new ache, fatigue and exceptional signs — even though it seems like they come and pass.

Fibromyalgia is a illness characterised through giant musculoskeletal ache discovered by fatigue, sleep, memory and temper troubles. Researchers agree with that fibromyalgia amplifies painful sensations by way of affecting the manner your brain and spinal cord process painful and nonpainful indicators.

Signs and symptoms often begin after an

event, such as bodily trauma, surgical treatment, infection or massive mental strain. In different instances, signs regularly gather over time and not using a unmarried triggering event.

Ladies are more likely to broaden fibromyalgia than are men. Many human beings who've fibromyalgia additionally have tension headaches, temporomandibular joint (TMJ) problems, irritable bowel syndrome, tension and depression.

At the same time as there may be no treatment for fibromyalgia, an expansion of medicinal drugs can help control signs. Exercising, rest and pressure-cut price measures additionally may additionally additionally help.

Fibromyalgia is a continual syndrome that could reason big frame ache, fatigue, and cognitive problems. Someone may additionally moreover confuse fibromyalgia signs and signs with those of arthritis, or joint infection.

Fibromyalgia is a continual (lengthy-term) disease described via pain and tenderness at some stage in your frame, in addition to fatigue.

Humans with fibromyalgia will be inclined to have a heightened experience of pain. This experience is every now and then defined as a regular muscle pain.

Fibromyalgia isn't a revolutionary disease, which means that it won't progressively worsen through the years.

There's no remedy for fibromyalgia, however treatments are to be had which can help relieve signs and symptoms and beautify your fine of lifestyles.

Who is laid low with fibromyalgia?

Certainly anyone can increase fibromyalgia. It influences human beings of any age, along with children. Round 4 million human beings within the U.S. Are living with fibromyalgia.

Human beings assigned lady at starting (AFAB) and people older than 40 are more likely to be diagnosed with fibromyalgia.

Signs

The number one signs and symptoms and symptoms of fibromyalgia encompass:

Large pain. The ache associated with fibromyalgia often is described as a constant stupid pain that has lasted for at the least 3 months. To be considered giant, the pain ought to arise on each aspects of your body and above and underneath your waist.

Fatigue. Humans with fibromyalgia regularly wake up tired, regardless of the reality that they record sleeping for lengthy intervals of time. Sleep is often disrupted with the useful resource of pain, and lots of sufferers with fibromyalgia have other sleep problems, which includes stressed legs syndrome and sleep apnea.

Cognitive difficulties. A symptom usually called "fibro fog" impairs the capability to focus, pay interest and deal with intellectual obligations.

Fibromyalgia regularly co-exists with exceptional conditions, which include:

Irritable bowel syndrome

Chronic fatigue syndrome

Migraine and other forms of headaches

Interstitial cystitis or painful bladder syndrome

Temporomandibular joint problems

Anxiety

Melancholy

Postural tachycardia syndrome

What reasons fibromyalgia?

Experts don't recognise what reasons fibromyalgia.

High quality genes you inherit from you natural dad and mom can also make you more likely to growth fibromyalgia. Research have discovered a link among organic dad and mom who've fibromyalgia and their youngsters — this could suggest it's handed down through families.

Humans with fibromyalgia are commonly greater sensitive to pain than most of the people. Experts haven't found the direct link but, however they suppose genetic mutations within the genes responsible for forming the neurotransmitters on your brain that broadcast and acquire ache indicators for your body may motive fibromyalgia.

What are the chance factors for fibromyalgia?

Even though specialists can't say for certain what motives fibromyalgia, a few health conditions and other problems are risk factors for growing it. Fibromyalgia chance elements embody:

Your age: people older than 40 are more likely to increase fibromyalgia. But it could have an effect on every body, together with youngsters.

Your sex assigned at begin: humans assigned woman at beginning are two instances as probably to enjoy fibromyalgia.

Continual illnesses: humans with situations like osteoarthritis, despair, anxiety disorders, chronic again pain and irritable bowel syndrome are much more likely to extend fibromyalgia.

Infections: some human beings broaden fibromyalgia after having an contamination, in particular if they experience extreme signs and symptoms.

Stress: the amount of strain you experience can't be measured on a take a look at, but too much pressure will have an impact to your fitness.

Traumas: folks who've skilled a physical or emotional trauma or a severe injury now and again increase fibromyalgia.

What triggers a fibromyalgia flare-up?

Nice occasions or adjustments to your life can cause a fibromyalgia flare-up. Each person is first rate, and what triggers symptoms and signs for a few humans won't for you. In general, something to be able to boom your strain can cause a flare-up, which encompass:

Emotional strain because of your mission, financial situation or social life.

Adjustments for your daily normal.

Adjustments to your eating regimen or now not getting sufficient vitamins.

Hormone changes.

Now not getting sufficient sleep or

converting whilst you sleep.

Climate or temperature modifications.

Getting sick.

Starting new remedy or remedies, or converting some issue for your regular fibromyalgia remedy habitual.

Complications

The pain, fatigue, and terrible sleep first-rate related to fibromyalgia can interfere together with your capability to characteristic at domestic or at the procedure. The frustration of coping with an frequently-misunderstood situation can also result in melancholy and fitness-associated anxiety.

CHAPTER TWO

How is fibromyalgia diagnosed?

A healthcare issuer will diagnose fibromyalgia with a physical examination and dialogue of your health history. They'll ask approximately your signs and while you first observed them.

There's no check that can diagnose fibromyalgia. Typically, diagnosing it's far part of a differential prognosis — a clinical technique of elimination. Your organisation will make a diagnosis by evaluating numerous situations with related signs. This procedure effects to your final evaluation.

Your employer may use blood checks to rule

out other commonplace reasons of fatigue like anemia or issues together together with your thyroid gland.

How is fibromyalgia handled?

There isn't a unmarried treatment that works for everybody with fibromyalgia. Your issuer will paintings with you to discover a aggregate of treatments that relieve your symptoms. Inform your company which signs and signs you're experiencing and once they trade (together with after they're enhancing or getting worse).

Remedies you could want encompass:

Over-the-counter (OTC) or prescription remedy to relieve ache.

Wearing sports like stretches or power training.

Sleep treatment.

Cognitive behavioral remedy.

Cognitive behavioral remedy (CBT) is a set up, purpose-oriented form of psychotherapy (speak therapy).

Mental health professionals, such as psychologists, therapists and counselors, use it to address or manipulate mental health situations and emotional concerns. It's one of the most commonplace and fantastic-studied forms of psychotherapy.

Psychological troubles are in component based on complicated or unhelpful types of thinking.

Intellectual troubles are in part based totally on discovered forms of unhelpful behavior.

Intellectual troubles are partly primarily based on complex middle ideals, together with critical thoughts approximately yourself and the world.

Human beings experiencing psychological troubles can studies better approaches of managing them. This will assist relieve their symptoms and enhance their intellectual and emotional fitness.

At some stage in CBT, a intellectual health professional permits you take a near study your mind and feelings. You'll come to apprehend how your thoughts have an effect on your movements. Thru CBT, you may unlearn horrible thoughts and behaviors and discover ways to undertake healthier questioning styles and behavior.

CBT typically takes place over a restricted amount of classes. The usage of a question-and-solution layout, your therapist facilitates you gain a particular mind-set. As a give up end result, you learn to reply higher to strain, ache and hard situations.

CBT can be used alone or in conjunction with medication and exclusive treatment alternatives. Your therapist will personalize your treatment primarily based totally on the problem you're addressing.

What situations can cognitive behavioral therapy (CBT) deal with?

Cognitive behavioral therapy is a precious device for treating and managing a extensive variety of intellectual health conditions and emotional demanding situations. People of every age (consisting of children) can obtain CBT.

Therapists and psychologists use CBT to treat many highbrow fitness situations, which incorporates:

Melancholy.

Tension.

Obsessive-compulsive disease (OCD).

Put up-worrying stress ailment (PTSD).

Interest-deficit/hyperactivity ailment (ADHD).

Phobias.

Character problems.

Eating troubles, collectively with bulimia, anorexia or binge consuming sickness.

Substance use disorder and alcohol use illness.

Even as mixed with treatment, CBT is useful in treating bipolar ailment and schizophrenia.

Studies have shown that CBT is likewise powerful in assisting manipulate nonpsychological scientific conditions, consisting of:

Insomnia.

Fibromyalgia and different reasons of persistent ache.

Continual fatigue syndrome.

Migraines.

Irritable bowel syndrome (IBS).

CBT can assist humans artwork thru regular worrying situations and life adjustments, too. You could are looking for help for troubles which includes:

Relationship issues.

Divorce.

Problems at artwork.

Grief.

Adjusting to a brand new life situation or clinical situation.

Pressure and coping troubles.

How do I find out a CBT therapist?

A therapist may be a psychologist, psychiatrist (a scientific physician who can prescribe drugs), psychiatric nurse, social employee or own family therapist.

Locating the proper therapist for you is usually a time-ingesting challenge. Attempt no longer to become discouraged. Talk to human beings you receive as true with to present you a referral for a therapist who makes use of cognitive behavioral treatment, whether it's your primary healthcare company or a friend or member of the family.

You could additionally look for therapists on line through nearby and country mental associations.

Ensure that any therapist you're interested by seeing is a country-certified and certified intellectual fitness expert and that they address your region of hassle (for instance, melancholy, eating troubles, substance use issues, and so forth.).

Maximum therapists' web web sites list the situations and problems they deal with. When you have questions, name or electronic mail the therapist's administrative center before you pick.

How does cognitive behavioral remedy (CBT) paintings?

Cognitive behavioral remedy is an evidence-primarily based treatment that's grounded in idea and capacity-primarily based completely communicate (conversations). It offers a supportive, nonjudgmental and safe surroundings that permits you to speak overtly with a mental fitness expert who's goal and in particular skilled that will help you with the issues you're having.

Cognitive behavioral treatment typically takes region over a limited quantity of periods (typically five to 20). You shouldn't expect results immediately. CBT commonly takes time and occasionally entails uncomfortable art work. Think about your therapist as a companion running with you via a process. If you preserve walking collectively in the path of the desires you've set, you'll be able to mark your development through the years.

Right right here's the way it works. Your therapist will:

Gain an understanding of the issue: on the start of remedy, you'll communicate stressful conditions you're managing, signs and symptoms and signs and symptoms you've located and any problems you have were given. In case you've been diagnosed with a mental health situation, inform your therapist. This important first step will help you region dreams to your remedy.

Ask a series of questions: relying in your scenario, your therapist might also ask you questions. You can talk an incident on your beyond, fears or phobias, troubling behaviors or your mind and emotions. Collectively, you'll discover your answers so that you can advantage belief into the way you reply to demanding situations on your existence.

Help you understand complicated mind and behaviors: via interactive question-and-answer lessons, your therapist will inspire you to pay close to attention to the way you reply to tough situations. You'll artwork collectively to turn out to be privy to horrific emotions, beliefs or behaviors that may be contributing to your problems. Your therapist can also ask you to preserve a magazine of these conditions and your responses to them.

Artwork with you to adjust your mind and behaviors: Your therapist will assist you locate tactics to exchange terrible emotions, thoughts and conduct. You can trade your mindset and adopt extremely good notion patterns and behaviors. Then, you may practice the ones skills to destiny situations.

What are the pros and cons of cognitive behavioral therapy (CBT)?

Cognitive behavioral therapy permits you end up more privy to your emotions, mind and behaviors. After CBT, most people adopt healthier conduct. CBT can't make disturbing situations disappear, but you can reply to them extra positively and feel higher usual.

Many studies display that CBT is as powerful as, or greater effective than, extraordinary types of mental treatment or psychiatric medicines.

Relying in your situation, you can sense slightly extra disillusioned during remedy. Your therapist will will let you artwork through those feelings. You could use new talents to triumph over poor emotions.

Stress manipulate therapy.

Stress is a normal human reaction that happens to everybody. In fact, the human body is designed to experience stress and react to it. At the same time as you enjoy changes or demanding situations (stressors), your frame produces physical and intellectual responses. That's stress.

CHAPTER THREE

Pressure responses help your body alter to new conditions. Stress may be amazing, preserving us alert, stimulated and organized to keep away from threat. For instance, if you have an essential take a look at arising, a pressure response might probable assist your body paintings extra difficult and stay awake longer. However pressure becomes a trouble at the same time as stressors keep with out remedy or durations of rest.

What takes place to the body in the course of pressure?

The body's autonomic nervous system controls your heart price, respiratory, vision adjustments and extra. Its built-in stress reaction, the "fight-or-flight reaction," enables the frame face disturbing conditions.

While a person has lengthy-term (persistent) pressure, persevered activation of the stress response reasons put on and tear on the frame. Bodily, emotional and behavioral signs and signs increase.

Physical symptoms of pressure encompass:

Aches and pains.

Chest pain or a feeling like your coronary heart is racing.

Exhaustion or trouble dozing.

Complications, dizziness or shaking.

High blood pressure.

Muscle anxiety or jaw clenching.

Belly or digestive troubles.

Hassle having sex.

Prone immune gadget.

Pressure can lead to emotional and mental signs like:

Tension or irritability.

Depression.

Panic assaults.

Sadness.

Consuming alcohol too much or too frequently.

Playing.

Overeating or developing an eating sickness.

Collaborating compulsively in sex, buying or internet surfing.

Smoking.

The use of pills.

How is stress identified?

Stress is subjective — no longer measurable with tests. Simplest the man or woman experiencing it can determine whether or now not it's far present and how immoderate it feels. A healthcare employer might also use questionnaires to recognize your strain and the way it affects your life.

When you have persistent stress, your healthcare company can examine symptoms and signs that stop result from stress. As an example, immoderate blood pressure can be identified and dealt with.

What are some techniques for stress remedy?

You could't keep away from pressure, however you may prevent it from turning into overwhelming with the aid of training some every day techniques:

Workout at the same time as you experience

symptoms of pressure approaching. Even a quick stroll can beautify your mood.

At the give up of every day, take a second to think about what you've finished — not what you didn't get accomplished.

Set desires to your day, week and month. Narrowing your view will help you experience extra on pinnacle of factors of the moment and lengthy-term responsibilities.

Take into account talking to a therapist or your healthcare company about your issues.

What are some approaches to save you stress?

Many each day techniques can help you preserve stress at bay:

Attempt relaxation sports, in conjunction with meditation, yoga, tai chi, respiratory physical sports and muscle relaxation. Programs are to be had on-line, in cellphone apps, and at many gyms and network centers.

Take properly care of your frame each day. Eating proper, exercise and getting enough sleep help your frame manipulate pressure a bargain higher.

Stay excessive first-class and practice gratitude, acknowledging the good components of your day or life.

Acquire that you may't manage the entirety.

Find out techniques to let bypass of worry approximately situations you can't alternate.

Examine to mention "no" to additional duties whilst you are too busy or pressured.

Stay linked with individuals who keep you calm, make you satisfied, provide emotional help and assist you with practical things. A chum, family member or neighbor can grow to be a awesome listener or percentage obligations so that stress doesn't turn out to be overwhelming.

How lengthy does stress last?

Pressure can be a quick-term difficulty or an extended-time period problem, relying on what changes for your lifestyles. Regularly the use of pressure management techniques can help you keep away from most physical, emotional and behavioral signs and symptoms of stress.

At the same time as need to I talk to a medical doctor approximately stress?

You have to are in search of for scientific interest in case you sense overwhelmed, in case you are the usage of pills or alcohol to cope, or when you have thoughts approximately hurting yourself. Your number one care agency can assist through imparting advice, prescribing remedy or referring you to a therapist.

What are the four levels of fibromyalgia?

Fibromyalgia is a dynamic situation. This

shows you gained't experience signs in any precise order — there's no roadmap to understand whilst or how fibromyalgia symptoms will have an effect on you.

Your company may deal with your fibromyalgia in degrees based totally on the way you experience. The ones tiers aren't a step-with the resource of-step treatment plan. All of us is unique, and how fibromyalgia affects your body can be precise. The degrees are extra like loose classes that can help you recognize which remedies you'll want to govern your signs and symptoms. The 4 ranges of treating fibromyalgia consist of:

Non-pharmacological treatments: Your issuer or a physical therapist will provide you with stretches and physical games to loosen, relax and make stronger your muscle businesses and joints.

Mental remedies: A mental health professional will assist you come to be privy to techniques to hold a wholesome self-image. They'll propose strategies to govern signs that have an effect to your intellectual and emotional health.

Pharmacological remedy: Taking remedy to control your signs.

Each day functioning: An occupational therapist permit you to navigate your day by day routine in case you're experiencing immoderate symptoms that make it tough to participate in your regular sports activities.

Because professionals don't recognize what motives fibromyalgia, you can't save you it.

Retaining your widespread health can help lessen the severity of fibromyalgia signs:

Manipulate stress similarly to you may.

Take a look at a weight loss plan and workout plan that's healthful for you.

Get sufficient sleep and exercise well sleep hygiene.

CONCLUSION

Fibromyalgia reasons pain all all through your frame. It may moreover make you revel in fatigued and like your mind is clouded with the useful resource of a fog. There's no treatment for fibromyalgia, but your healthcare issuer will help you find out a mixture of remedies that relieve your signs and symptoms.

Notwithstanding the truth that experts don't understand what reasons fibromyalgia, it's real — and so are your signs. They will come and pass or be tough to describe, however how you feel is legitimate and important. Residing with a continual situation like fibromyalgia may be a mission, but you don't ought to do it by myself. Talk for your organisation or a mental health expert about coping with pressure and keeping a powerful self-photograph.

THE END